Codependency Cure for the Soul

Steps to Break Free from Addiction, Abuse, Trauma and Enable Healthy Relationships Conquering your Emotional Health and Happiness

Table of Contents

Introduction

There are many people who don't know the difference between being in a healthy relationship and being in one that is codependent. However, if you can answer these questions honestly, it will give you a clue about whether your relationships are healthy or whether you need to reappraise them and adjust your own behavior so that you can live your life peacefully and happily away from codependence:

- Are you the type of person to keep quiet rather than argue the point?
- Are you concerned about the opinion that people have of you?
- Does life make you feel inadequate?
- Do you feel used up sometimes?
- Are you confused about where your life is going?

Unfortunately, all of these are signs of codependence. They mean that you haven't yet made your mark on your life or taken ownership of it. You have simply gone from one unsatisfactory situation to the next without being able to control the situation. You may even see it as being the fault of someone else. You may also doubt that you will ever feel fulfilled by life and may have given up on the idea of your own importance.

The problem with this kind of relationship in life is that it takes the front seat and your life gets stacked away in the back seat. Thus, you have no control over where life is taking you. You simply go along with it because you see this as your only solution. This book delves into why people feel this inadequacy and depend upon relationships that are at best unsatisfactory and at worst, positively abusive. You don't need to be hit on a regular basis to be abused. However, when you let someone else dictate the course of your life, based upon their own unrealistic view point, you may as well package your life into a box and give it away. Codependent people do that. When you read through this book, you will find solutions.

You will be able to see the steps that you need to take to move out of this negative situation and have the confidence to walk forward in your life under your own steam. Of course, love may be involved, but that doesn't mean that you need to lie down and be someone's doormat. Quite often, people deny the situation because it's easier than admitting to unhappiness. However, the fact that you are reading this introduction to the book tells me that you have questions about forming adequate relationships to make your life a better place to be.

Through the exercises shown in the book, you will find that your self-esteem will soar and that you will have a better view of what's going on in your world and be able to make decision based – not upon the wishes of others – but upon your own common sense and your need to assert your views and your own values. When you leave the ranks of the codependent, you become happier and are able to see yourself as whole. That's the aim of this book. Codependency weakens you and takes you away from your own core values to please others who may not merit that attention. If you feel that you need help in this direction, then this book is written in no-nonsense terms to help you see through the fog toward the light of day. Walk with me along this path and let me guide you toward discovering who you really are. You have so much value in this life that you have yet to unleash and that's the only reason for writing this book.

Having worked with people in codependent relationships for the past 15 years, it is my intention that you learn to understand that life can be changed and that you, with my help, can live to enjoy your life and to fulfill your own dreams. They matter and should always matter, regardless of what demands others impose upon you. I hope that in some small way this book will help you to see the trap that you are in and why you are in it, because, in order to move forward, you need to learn how to maximize your life's value and conquer the need for people who sap your energy and your time. What all readers need to understand is that codependency is certainly not an illness. It is something that can be combatted, once the behavior is broken down and understood.

Assessment Test - Codependency

It is possible to assess the level of codependency and there are rather a lot of tests that you can find online. Here are some typical questions that you will be asked to see whether you are indeed codependent:

Do you make sacrifices to keep your relationship on track?
YES/NO

Have relationships contributed to your happiness?
YES/NO

Have your relationships ever affected the way other people see you?   YES/NO

Has your ambition in life changed since getting into this relationship? YES/NO

Do you often stay in a relationship longer than you should?
YES/NO

Have you ever borrowed money to finance your partner's addiction?   YES/NO

Have you ever felt that things you do are not recognized by others?   YES/NO

Do you stop buying things you need to avoid arguments?
YES/NO

Do you have difficulty sleeping at night because of your relationship? YES/NO

Have you ever wished that a loved one could see things your way?   YES/NO

Have you ever considered self-harm as a result of your relationship?   YES/NO

If most of your answers to the above questions are YES, then you are probably codependent and need to work through the chapters of this book to help yourself to see beyond codependency. There is a better life waiting for you and it takes making a few adjustments to the way that you see life. Don't worry. I am aware of how painful this is and the steps that are included in the chapters that follow will be small steps that you can take safely so that you work toward improving your self-esteem and personal strength. This will lead to being able to fix your relationship or at least being able to see it from a more reasoned viewpoint, so that you can make choices in your life that benefit you rather than detracting from your own importance. Even if your codependency has happened as a result of your childhood, it is not too late to modify your behavior and to change your approach. The most common feeling that codependent people experience is anxiety. This is why the book deals with codependency in a gentle way so that you have nothing to be afraid of, as you find your way back to understanding that your priorities need to change.

Chapter One: What is Codependency?

If you find yourself in a relationship with someone who you consider to be more important than you, you may be codependent. This isn't the only sign and there are several types of codependence. Often associated with relationships with addicts, alcoholics or even relationships between caregivers and abusive people, codependency is when you put another person before yourself to an extent that you suffer, but find it hard to break out of the cycle of what other people may consider to be abuse of some kind.

The amount of sacrifice you are prepared to give to that person is unreasonable and usually you put yourself in second place and may also suffer from self-esteem issues. A psychologist at California Polytechnic State University describes the relationship between the codependent and others as perhaps stemming from childhood experiences and that unreasonable expectations of the child can lead to unreasonable performance as an adult. These are people who depend upon a relationship that is skewed in favor of the abuser and yet codependent people will bend their own routines and lifestyle to fit that of the person to whom they are dependent.

This kind of relationship can happen in a couple, in a parent child situation and even in a work situation at different levels, though the main basis for its unhealthiness is that the codependent person puts him/herself last and does not see that there is anything wrong with doing so. These are people who put aside their own physical and mental wellbeing to support someone they feel they cannot exist without.

Psychologists say that it is possible to mend a codependent relationship by coming up with boundaries that suit both parties although most codependents are anxious and may be afraid of losing that one person they depend so heavily upon by creating waves. Another way to deal with codependency is the gradual widening of social interaction although this is not always the best solution, particularly if the social circle is only of the abuser's friends and family, in which case the codependent person may feel isolated or overwhelmed.

Chapter Two: Evaluating Self

I once asked a patient why she allowed others to walk all over her. She looked at me blankly. For the past ten years, she had been married to a man who drank too much and who came home regularly and treated her in an unreasonable manner. It was her who was seeking treatment, rather than him, although she saw herself as not being able to cope anymore and having no personal strength. She had truly had enough. She looked back at me and her answer was that she thought that other people mattered more than she did. Over the years of abuse, she truly had become worn down and persuaded by her abuser that she had no value without him. He made her feel like she could never survive on her own and because she loved him, she believed him.

The trouble with these kinds of thoughts are that they are borne from the abuse that comes with codependency. If you asked someone who was happy and independent if that person would put up with the kind of treatment that the lady in our example did, the answer would usually be "no" while for codependent people, this is an everyday scenario that is as natural to them as breathing.

When you evaluate your relationships, there are two criteria that you need to ask yourself in order to evaluate your role in life. These are:

- Does this friend give as much to the relationship as I do?

- Does my partner love who I am or constantly put me down?

You need to write down a list of your relationships and that can include work colleagues, friends and family and all those who have an influence in your life and decide which category they belong to. If you find that the majority use you and that you let them or that people put you down and make you feel less important, then you need to examine your life to find out what it is about you that makes people react in this manner. Not everyone has lives that are dictated by others, but most people who are codependent do. There may be strong connections between why you feel so bad and the people who you associate with negativity in your life.

There's another list you also need to make and that is of the people who respect you, who give you love or friendship and who don't use you. These are healthy relationships and should be fostered more than those who make you feel negative about yourself. By surrounding yourself with unhappy relationships, you add to the self-esteem issues and see yourself as having no value. The lady in the above example did just that and in her notes, what was apparent was that she had been bossed around for most of her life. She came from a dysfunctional family and most of her childhood, had been expected to take second place to her mother's new husband. As she grew older, she got into a relationship as a means of escape from home. The problem was that her self-esteem was already low.

If your self-esteem is low, the kind of people you attract into your life are likely to be those who can easily take advantage of your generosity and continue the cycle of abuse that you are accustomed to. Our example went through various relationships and ended up with a husband whose use of alcohol was excessive and whose use of violence to solve household issues was well known. She had attended hospital several times and had never admitted to staff that her bruises and broken bones were anything other than clumsiness on her part.

Evaluate your situation. Your husband may not beat you. Your wife may not be violent, but if either have the effect of cutting your importance down and making you feel less than whole, it isn't exactly a loving and tender way for someone to treat you. I know that your love for this person may have been the hurdle you always had when trying to break loose from a codependent relationship but it's time to make a stance and decide here and now that you can't take any more and start working on increasing your own sense of worth, so that you no longer depend upon people who diminish your value.

That doesn't necessarily mean divorce. These situations can be worked through, though you have to want to move forward and show your true colors instead of hiding behind the fear of letting abusers know what your true feelings are and realizing that you do have a right to an opinion. We need to build up your self-esteem levels so that you can eventually say, "Enough is enough" and let the future decide which way fate takes you. While you continue to allow people to use you, to disappoint you and to make false promises that always lead to disappointment, you can never really be happy, because your happiness as a codependent person is placed firmly in the hands of people who do not merit that level of trust.

Chapter Three: Recapturing your Small Ambitions

In this step of the process, you already know that your relationships are not satisfactory. Nothing is going to change overnight. However, you need to start keeping a journal of all the ideas you ever had about what you want to do with your life. The idea of this is to get back all of the dreams and ambitions that may have been denied you up until now. Here is a short list of the kind of things that can be on the kind of list I have in mind. Your wishes should not be based upon anything that anyone else influences you in. Your list should be strictly the things that you thought you would have liked to do as you grew up, but that life seems to have denied you until this point in time.

- I want to go walking at weekends
- I want to play tennis
- I want to listen to my favorite music
- I want to have my favorite flowers in the house
- I want to go out with my buddies once a week
- I want to enjoy nature more often

You are probably denied much of this because you don't have time to devote to you. However, whether you are a man or a woman, I want you to use this list as your wish list and over the next month, choose something on that list and do it, regardless of what other people dictate to you. For example, an abusive wife may stop you from going out with friends. An abusive husband may never pander to your wish to listen to the music you love.

There's no reason why you cannot try for the things that are attainable and make them something to wake up for each day. If you think that going out with buddies is pushing your luck too far, how about being able to have a family barbecue with friends? That means that you get to choose who comes and take the lead with preparations. Your list is private and personal and no one can dictate what your dreams are. These are very basic changes that won't put you at risk and you do need to exert your personal power to make some of them happen.

If you have trouble envisioning anything that you want to do, close your eyes and try to remember those things that presented you with happy moments in your life. See the people you were with, in your mind's eye, and see the situation as if it was happening right now. This helps you to go back to a time when you were happier and can be your secret place to go when you find that you are overwhelmed by life. One of my clients used to play the piano. This had long since stopped, but she remembered sitting at the piano and seeing herself as a concert pianist. This helped her as a child to get through her classes and excel at putting emotion into her music. The glint in her eye as she described this action was enough to be able to see that the experience was probably one of the happiest in her life. By using this experience to brighten up days when life offered her very little, she was able to introduce some positivity into her life. When you use visualization, you are able to switch off this moment which may be troubling you and step into another place and time to experience that happiness that makes your life feel it's worth something.

You will be given other exercises that are not as escapist as this, but for the time being until you build up your self-confidence and esteem, this exercise can help you move away from fear and the feeling of having no significance. You do have significance and you need to introduce it into your life each day to help affirm that you are an individual in your own right and have the right to your own dreams. If you find it hard to find the time to use this exercise, put aside time when you are alone. Even if this is in the cloakroom or in the privacy of the shower, you can close your eyes and be there, whenever life is making you feel there's not much in it for you. Be important, build up the image that makes you feel happy inside your heart and be assured that the steps within this book will help you to reach a stage in your life when this feeling of happiness will be more frequent.

Recap of exercises in this chapter

Make a list of things you always wanted to do. These shouldn't be bucket list items because it may not be possible to do such things at the moment. Make them relatively small things that you can introduce so that more of your time is devoted to your own pleasure. It's important, because it helps you to build up your self-esteem.

Then use the experience of visualization to pinpoint times in your life that gave you a lot of personal pleasure. These are items that are personal to you, rather than to you and someone else. Thus don't let the way your life has been dictated by others to decide the items you visualize. These need to be yours. Try to see an experience in your life that filled you with some kind of happiness and use this as your escape from negative thoughts when you are alone. Even people within abusive relationships who are codependent need to break free sometimes, even if initially only for a very short time each day.

Chapter Four: Codependency in the Workplace

Have you ever felt put upon in the workplace? Yet you still volunteer to help out when there is something that needs doing in a hurry. The problem may be codependency but it may not be adding to your career prospects. No matter how hard you work and how much work you produce, if you are codependent upon a boss who uses you, the chances are that you also play a part in the situation. People who lack confidence and who seek approval for the work that they do are often codependent without realizing it. When they don't receive praise of any kind, they go out of their way to seek it. This doesn't make you a valuable member of staff, even though you may see yourself as being indispensable. You may even find that you are taken for granted so much that even when you take a vacation, you come back to all the work piled up ready for you.

In a situation such as this, you are being used because you allow yourself to be used. You may not see it that way and may crave the approval that you have. However, it's unlikely that you will be considered for promotion, because your needy nature means that you don't have what it takes to be management material. It may sound like a bit of a downer to you that you have worked so hard for little return, but you are placing yourself in a very vicious circle and need to break free of it. Not only that, you may also be someone who prefers to work alone and are not a particularly good team member. You don't know how to delegate and would rather be weighed down with work and feel needed than share what you have with others.

This is a situation that will eventually lead to burn out and although people may have warned you about that, your nature won't make you believe it. You do what you do because perhaps you don't get praise in any other area of your life. You need to appraise your life and decide upon the following:

- Do you have a good work life/home life balance?
- Do you enjoy the work that you do?
- Would you enjoy it as much without the praise that you seek?

To get out of the vicious circle that you have put yourself in for some reason or other, you need to look back into your past and find out at what stage of your life you first felt that you were not given recognition for something that you did, because often this type of codependence stems from childhood.

Linda knew that she had problems but she didn't know how serious they were. Every day she dutifully went to work and slaved although no one had ever expected that amount of devotion from an employee in a relatively junior position. The problem arose when she suddenly realized during the absence of her boss that no one else seemed to give her the kind of feedback she craved. She was lost. Then, looking through her past with a therapist, what she found was that during her childhood, her mother never recognized anything that she did as being worthwhile. Her mother would even leave the room rather than acknowledge that Linda could do something that her mother was incapable of. All the years of childhood, she had tried her best to impress her mother – not because she needed to – but because she felt displaced and even had doubts about whether her mother was really her mother. She couldn't understand why her mother could not acknowledge her. This followed her into adulthood and in her first job, she was surprised that people actually thought what she was doing was a worthwhile job. Then she questioned their sincerity in her own mind, believing herself not really to be worthy of the praise that she was getting. Thus the cycle began and she craved that feedback that only her boss could give her.

The problem with this type of behavior is that she didn't actually need that acknowledgement and was quite capable of doing a good day's work but had slipped into the need for it feeling that it was the only thing that validated her. If you feel that you are falling into this trap at work, you need to find a new way forward because it is neither healthy nor productive to be so dependent upon someone else to validate who you are. A boss who wants more and more out of you may actually encourage weak people to do more and more work because usually people with low self-esteem don't ask much in return for their work. Often feeling validated is every bit as important as getting a fair pay for a good day's work.

Exercises related to work based codependency

While it may not be the healthiest thing for you to give up your job, especially if you count on it to pay your bills, you need to take a different approach. Observe people around you and see how they cope with the workload that they have. If you don't ask for validation, the only validation you really need is from yourself. If you know that you did a great day's work, learn not to ask for validation. Instead of that, treat yourself to something and congratulate yourself for what you have done. In Linda's case, she learned to do things to please herself. You must do the same. Inside of you, you have something called motivation. Don't let it be controlled by someone else. Control it yourself and you become motivated without needing insincerity and wasting the time seeking it. Most of the time, abusive bosses pile on more work when you seek this kind of validation and you end up feeling overwhelmed instead of pleased that you were able to manage your workload.

Don't do it for him or her. Do it for you. Set small goals for yourself that no one else knows about. People who always try come out as winners. Believe me, it takes a while for this to sink in but it really does work. For example, if you have a dozen tasks to do in a day, work out which ones take priority and set yourself little targets that are doable. Gain your confidence within yourself by keeping to your own timetable. Of course, priority jobs get done first, but you need to switch the motivation. It's not for the boss. It's for you. Make the competition inside yourself sufficiently motivating that when you succeed at something, only you know about it. What other people know about your skills and your goals is inconsequential at the end of the day.

By doing this, you build up confidence in yourself and don't need validation from anyone. In Linda's case, she was a brilliant artist, but because her mother had never acknowledged it, she had put away her paintbrushes and had given up on her passion in life. No one should ever let someone else dictate their success. When she finally built up her reputation as a brilliant painter, she did so on her own terms and people were quick to ask her to do drawings for them. In fact, she had no trouble making her passion into something quite substantial, although she also learned that she didn't have to please someone else as long as she was happy with the results. She also learned to say "no" which is a very hard lesson for someone who has self-esteem and codependency issues.

Exercise 2 – Setting yourself free

Give yourself some personal goals as well as work related goals and make them manageable. The reason you start simple is so that you can attain those goals. Then, little by little, as you gain confidence, you can make the goals a little harder. Remember that you are only creating them for yourself and for no one else. You are the only one that you are out to please. When you have made your goals for at home and you have kept them, look at your face in the mirror and see yourself as the success that you are. At the end of the day, the only person's opinion of you that matters is your own. When you can acknowledge your own successes, you don't need to be dependent upon your boss to validate you and you can go forward in your career because you are no longer a drain on people.

Chapter Five – Volunteerism

In this chapter, I want you to meet Anne Marie. She was codependent to the extent that she felt that she had very little significance at all. It was hard to persuade her that she had value. In fact, she had been codependent most of her life. When I introduced her to volunteerism, she hadn't realized what a difference it would make to her life. When you learn to give with absolutely no expectation of return or praise, you trigger something inside your brain that helps you to see your own value.

In the last chapter, I talked about how good it feels inside to achieve something just because you set yourself a goal. In this chapter, I want to take that feeling a step further. You are going to be feeling good simply because you did something good. In Anne Marie's case, she volunteered at the local dog shelter to help with stray dogs. She fed them, she groomed them and she took them for walks twice a week. It doesn't matter how often you do something like this. What matters is that you approach this work with a certain attitude.

"I am doing this because it pleases me to do it."

When you approach life in this manner, you give without expecting anything in return. Anne Marie's mother gave her a private education with strings attached and what this meant was that her mother expected Anne Marie to be forever grateful for what her mother had sacrificed for her. Her mother decided which kind of work Anne Marie did. She decided what kind of man Anne Marie would marry and lessened the importance of Anne Marie having any kind of opinion at all.

Introducing volunteerism in its truest form helped her to see that there were not always strings attached. When you give, you give through wanting to be of service, not because you expect something to happen as a result of your giving – like her mother had done. Anne Marie walked the dogs and soon came to realize how much the dogs looked forward to her visit. She began to feel light hearted and joyful for the first time that she could ever remember and I explained why.

When you give with no expectations at all, the reward that you feel is an inner reward. You go about your life humble in your approach, but when you give, you have a warm feeling inside that tells you that you have value. You don't need anyone's validation. You don't need to tell the world that you did something nice. You simply did it. That makes you better than those who give with strings attached.

Exercise for this chapter

For this chapter's exercise, I want you to do something for someone else without them having to ask you and do it with all the goodness of your heart, expecting nothing in return. This could be something simple like baking a cake for a friend or for the old lady who lives down the road. When asked why you did it, you simply need to say, "Because I wanted to." The feeling that you will get inside is one that will help to build up your self-esteem. It makes you feel better inside and that's what it's all about. It's a very simple gesture, but it teaches you the power you have to change your view of the world.

Volunteering can take any form whatsoever and what it does is help you to help yourself to feel better about life. If you give with expectations of thanks or gratitude, forget it. Give because you want to give. You set yourself up for disappointment if you do it because you care about what other people think. When you do it for you, you allow yourself to live life on your terms and it doesn't matter if people are ungracious. That's their problem, rather than being yours. The kind of things that you can volunteer for are shown below:

- Serve soup at a soup kitchen once a week
- Help at a homeless shelter
- Help in a shelter for dogs
- Help at the local school
- Help at the local center for seniors
- Do nice things for people you know

If you do choose to do nice things for people you know, make sure it's for the right motives. You are not seeking approval. You are merely doing something because you choose to. When you wake up in the morning, ask yourself what you can do today for someone else and what you can do for yourself. Both of these activities help you to build your self-esteem.

Chapter Six: Learning to Say, "No"

This is one of the hardest things for someone who is codependent. They generally go along with whatever is suggested, even when it is to their detriment. However, you need to be able to stand up for yourself. Perhaps you are in a situation where people take you for granted and, up until now, you have allowed this to happen. You need to learn to say no in a way that cannot be misconstrued though you may have to break into this kind of activity gently. You won't be accustomed to it and if you think yourself less important than others, you tend to oblige them because it's your way of getting validation. You don't need this kind of validation. Little do you know, people are thinking how easy you are to persuade and are actually viewing you as a doormat. You need to halt that practice and here are a few phrases that you can use where you won't offend too much:

"I am sorry, I am busy tonight."

"I am so sorry. I have too much on my plate at the moment."

"I can't help you this time as I have other obligations."

You don't need to be rude about it, but you do need to stop letting people walk over you. Let me tell you the case of Nancy. Nancy would make birthday cakes for people but she loved having their validation all of the time and wouldn't say no to anyone even if she knew she was short of time. She ended up staying up half the night to make cakes and could see that she was gradually wearing herself out. It wasn't a business. She got nothing for doing the cakes, but her codependency was upon the people around her who kept letting her know what a great person she was and feeding off her vulnerability.

She broke down in tears as she explained her situation. She was afraid that if she said "No" she would lose her friends. Nancy never really changed much because she didn't listen to the advice she was given. When she died at the age of 65, the church was empty except for her daughter. None of those friends who had used her all of her life came to bid her farewell. I am telling you this story because it is shocking and because those people who use others wear down your self-esteem but are never there when you need something in return. That's not friendship and the fact that you continue to do things for people like this shows your own weaknesses and codependency. The relationships are not healthy when they are one-sided and most of the people who demand one-sided relationships give nothing at all in exchange and are not of value long term.

Exercise for this chapter

I want you to say "no" to someone. It may be someone who asks you to do things rather a lot, but you do need to sort out one thing first. Work out which relationships are two way. You will know which people are truly kind to you and go out of their way to help you but you will also know the people you dread phoning you because you know that their phone calls always include some kind of demand of your time. These are the people you need to say "no" to. It could be your boss asking you to overtime yet again or it could be someone who asks you to babysit or to pick up their kid from school. If it means that you need to go out of your way to do whatever it is that they ask of you, think up a suitable reply in the negative:

"I am sorry, I am going out this afternoon."

"I am sorry, I have a friend coming round."

"I can't because I am already overloaded."

"I can't work overtime this weekend. I have guests coming."

The first time that you say no, you will worry about it. Don't back down. Once you do this on an ongoing basis to people who give nothing in return for your friendship, then it frees up time for you to do the things that you want to do. It also helps you to prioritize your time in a much better way. Each time that you are able to say "no" think of something you can do that you enjoy doing instead of doing whatever it was that they asked you to do. Get a life. Do the things YOU want to do and start feeling good about it. Whether it means treating yourself to a massage or simply having an afternoon viewing of a movie you love, your time is yours to do with as you please, rather than always having it taken up by doing things for other people.

Phone a true friend. Visit your family or simply go out window shopping. It doesn't matter what it is that you do as long as it's something for yourself. It's not selfish. It is giving you back your self-respect and upping your self-esteem by putting yourself first for a change. Happy people attract happy people and when you get over being used by people, and start to look after your own interests, you come into contact with other positive people who will enhance your life by appreciating you for who you are.

Chapter Seven: Caregiving versus Caretaking

When you are persuaded to act in a way that you don't want to, you are being manipulated. Those to whom you are codependent are very good at manipulating you and you never really see it in that way. You see it as simply being in a relationship with that person.

Caregivers versus Caretakers

Look at the behaviors below and test yourself to see which category you fall into. Are you a caregiver or are you a caretaker?

Caretaker	Caregiver
May feel stressed by having to care and sharing love	Enjoys caring
Caretakers have no boundaries boundaries	Respect
Gives with strings attached	Gives freely
Attract needy people	Attract healthy people

Those who are in a position where the relationship causes them stress and expectations will find that they are often unfulfilled and unhappy. Cross that line toward becoming a caregiver, and you are able to give more freely because you are not expecting returns and are doing so because you want to. Earlier in the book I talked about doing something just because you want to because it is vital that you understand the codependence as opposed to the relationship you form with someone by simply wanting to give.

In the scenario in the office, if you feel codependent upon an abusive boss, similarly, you will feel obligation rather than wanting to perform the job to the best of your ability for yourself.

All relationships that are codependent have something in common. You need to recognize that they have the following elements in common:

- Pressure
- Unwillingness
- Dread
- Fear

Thus, these are the traits you need to overcome to step away from codependence. In the next chapter, I will show you how to step beyond these boundaries that you have placed upon your life and to do so in such a way that you can hold your head up high and feel that you have acted in an appropriate way. When you are codependent, you find it hard to say "no" and you also find it hard to raise your own self-esteem and will always place the needs of others before yourself. This is something you need to get out of the habit of doing because each time you give way to codependency, you step one step further away from independence and being able to enjoy life on your own terms.

Exercise for this chapter

Work out what things you do in your life that make you feel forced to do as opposed to wanting to do. Work out how you feel when you do these things. Are you a caregiver or a caretaker? On whose terms do you live your life?

Now write down some boundaries and do not be afraid to introduce them. For example, if the person to whom you are codependent asks too much of you, write down what you would do for that person willingly. Draw up boundaries and share them with that person but make sure that you keep to them. These can include such things as:

- I will only work 5 days a week
- I will only work between these hours
- My room is private and should not be entered

You can make your own boundaries that suit your situation. Don't be afraid to stick to them. If you are caring for an elderly relative, make other arrangements to fit in with yours. There are care agencies. You don't have to take on the whole load yourself. In fact, if you do, you are automatically going to give less and begrudge more. You need to get your life back and stop allowing yourself to be used.

Chapter Eight: Boundaries

Some people who are codependent go beyond what is called for to cater to the anxiety of the person to whom they are codependent. They try to fix things before they are broken. They attempt to lay emphasis on the person they are dependent upon. They will use the word "you" more than "I" and there's a very good reason. They consider themselves to be unimportant. Say, for example, the codependent person is married to a drunk. Their acceptance level of their partner's behavior may be totally unreasonable to normal people and they are made to feel shame when they don't live up to their partner's expectations. Shame is something that works on the subconscious and is translated as self-defeating or cutting down the importance of an individual. The drunk's wife is made to feel shame because she didn't get the dinner ready for the return of her husband, even though he is three hours late. The problem with this kind of shame is that builds up and when you feel built up shame, you don't tend to differentiate between shame and guilt.

Let's look at the core differences between guilt and shame, so that you can see if your thoughts are based upon what's happening to you or to someone you are codependent upon.

Guilt

You are able to judge behavior

You fear being punished

Leads you to self-improvement

Doesn't lead to shame if resolved

Shame

You judge yourself

You fear being abandoned

Leads to anger and aggression

Causes low self-esteem

Thus, someone who feels guilt would have normal and rational fears whereas someone who feels shame will not respond to situations in the normal way. They will feel that they lack importance and will see every flaw as adding to their inadequacy. If you are in an unhealthy codependent relationship, this may be furthered by your abuser affirming that you are useless, that you don't have intelligence and that you measure short of normal. This is their way of controlling the situation. As long as you feel shame, you will not seek the help of others because to do so will humiliate you and you see humiliation and shame as being one and the same thing.

I want you to keep a journal and when something happens that makes you feel shame or humiliation, write down what triggered it and examine it thoroughly. Why did you feel shame and was what happened really your fault? Be honest and think with the mind distanced from the situation. Was there something that you could have done to make the outcome satisfactory? Was there something to learn from the situation which would stop you from making the same mistake again? If there was, then the shame you are feeling is normal.

Now I want you to draw a diagram. There are several circles, one inside the other. The central circle is **THE REAL YOU.** That may not surface much these days. The next circle is **the**

devalued you. That means when you are feeling a state of shame. The third circle is **the observer**. This is the person you become when you evaluate the situation honestly to see where fault lies. The next circle represents your **character or the persona** of you. The outside circle is all about **the ideal you**. When something happens that is negative consequences, examine each circle in turn and find out why there are negative consequences. Let me give you an example.

Sara allows her husband to walk all over her and today he threw the washing on the floor and asked her to pick it up. Why did she do it? If she looks at her chart of circles, she may find that the real Sara in the center of the chart is basically tidy. Although she feels she picked it up because of fear of consequence, she also did it because she is fundamentally tidy but has no boundaries in place that lets her husband know his behavior is unreasonable. In actual fact, she can see clearly that the fault lies with her husband when she looks at the situation through the observer circle. She picked up the washing because it is her persona to be tidy. Thus, she feels that her ideal was reached by doing what she did.

Nowadays, since she is no longer codependent, she has set up boundaries and if her husband crosses those boundaries, she has learned not to respond. She placed these boundaries upon her relationship when her mind was clear and her husband was calm. "I have children to clear up after and I will not clean up after you if you make a mess." As her husband was remorseful about his treatment of her, she was able to use this time to establish a boundary that he respected her for.

Exercise for this chapter

Keep a note of situations that annoyed you or made you feel ashamed or humiliated by the person who whom you are codependent. Use the diagram to work out the logic of the situation in retrospect. Now, work out a boundary you can set to take you away from situations such as this, and stick to those boundaries.

Examples:

If you treat me like a slave I will not respond.

You should hang up your own clothing.

I will make coffee in the morning but it would be nice if you make coffee in the evening.

The thing that you need to do is to swing the balance so that instead of doing things just because someone else wants you to, you get to do things because you actually see them as being things you want to do within the guidelines that you set. For example, if you are looking after an elderly person, you must distance yourself sometimes. You do need to have time off and there are agencies that help to give people in your situation some respite. The kind of boundaries that you can set up in this case would be:

I will leave the commode within easy reach of the bed and the light on

I am taking Friday's off each week

I am looking forward to my program on the TV tonight at 8

You have to show that you have respect for your own wishes. That doesn't mean getting involved in conflict. It just means that you do need to start to care for your own interests because while you are doing all these things for others and making them more important than you, you are doing nothing to re-establish your own self-esteem and that's extremely important. When you set boundaries, you are able to deal with your duties in a much more positive way and actually get to enjoy any obligation that you have without having to dread the interaction. You give yourself a little bit of time and during this time, make sure that you do something that pleases you.

Chapter Nine: Recovery from Codependence

In the last chapter, I discussed the diagram with circles and you should use this to help you to decide on whether you are being authentic in your life or not, Remember, the inner circle represents your True Self. However, your true self is forever changing depending upon the way that you live your life. Although the core you doesn't change, your attitudes change with time. The next circle is the devalued self and this is where you currently are. You don't feel like you have that much value and you feel like you don't have much choice in your life, but that's where you are wrong. If you use the third circle and evaluate situations, you can learn from them and move on from codependency so that you come out as the Ideal person you would like to be.

The word ideal is very subjective. One person wants one thing and another gets joy from other things. To help you to see what you get joy from, I would like you to sit down and write down the things you are grateful for each day because these will help you to evaluate your position from a more positive perspective. Read through your list of gratitude each day before you attempt to make yourself feel positive about who you are. Then, look at any situation that is giving you problems and work out the different scenarios which can lead to you becoming the ideal person. Let's show you an example,

You have a lot of housework to do today. You feel overwhelmed. You also know that there won't be enough money to pay the bills this month.

This is your true situation at this moment in time. What can you do to change it?

1) Get the housework done quickly so you have more time for yourself.
2) Decide to set yourself a goal and keep it as far as the housework is concerned.
3) Do the jobs that you know will be noticed.
4) Look at your true financial situation so you are not worried about something that really isn't that bad.
5) Work out ways that you can save a little to help you to pay your bills.
6) Think about others much worse off who don't even have a roof over their heads.
7) Think how lucky you are to have a home.

You need to work out your own answers to your own problems in life, but you need to come to decisions that help you to be less codependent and more independent. For example, Nicole was in exactly the same situation as described above. She always saw herself as unimportant. Her first priority was her husband who was a drug addict. Everything went on his habit. She had no money left. What she didn't see was that it was possible to pay the bills simply by cutting something else out of her spending. She was a very good cook and managed to make delicious meals on a very tight budget and put away enough money so that the bills could be paid without her husband knowing that she had skimped. She actually started to enjoy the cooking process and gained a lot of satisfaction from the independence it gave her as well as being able to share this with her husband. As far as the housework was concerned, she gave herself a set time within which to do the housework so that she had time left over for herself. That was a rarity. How she did this was to tell herself that what wasn't finished by a set time would be left to another day. She set goals for urgent things and did these, but actually surprised herself at doing more than she planned.

Every day you get challenges. Every day you get a chance to tackle life in a better way that gives you more and there's nothing wrong with taking that time for you. You need to build up your friendships. You need to find that ideal self that lies in the outside circle and when you do, you begin to feel stronger and more positive about yourself. While you are codependent, you tend to put your own needs on the back shelf and that's never going to contribute to happiness. You will end up resenting what you feel forced to do with your life though it's only your codependence that forces you. If you build up your own self-esteem by allowing yourself a little bit of enjoyment – regardless of the circumstances you are in – you can actually give your loved one more because happiness counts. Happy people give more. Look at the friendships you have with happy people and what you find is that you don't dread their visits. You don't feel bad about their positivity. When you are happy, people will feel like that about you as well.

Only you can help yourself in this situation. Of course, there are counselors who are expert in this field, but this book is all about YOU and what YOU can do on your own to help you to regain the following:

- Pride in yourself
- Happiness in your heart
- Gratitude for your life
- Love for yourself

The thing that you may not realize is that codependency wrecks lives and it's not just your life that is being wrecked. It is toxic and changes your overall view of life and your relationships and breeds so much regret, unhappiness and bitterness. By learning to love yourself, you move on and are able to live a happier life and thus give more to your friends and family than you ever could while you hold onto the need to please others. Step off the roundabout that is destroying your life and begin to see beyond it.

I want you to go back to chapter two and look at the exercise there where you have to decide the small things that you want to do in your life. These can be miniscule steps. They don't have to be huge things. Maybe you deprive yourself of things because you feel you don't deserve them. Its nonsense, but it's what you believe. Now is the time to break free from that slavery. Stop doing it to yourself and make sure that every day, you do at least one thing that is your choice. It could be something as simple as:

- Treating myself to a peach
- Washing my hair and using a conditioner
- Dressing in my nice clothes
- Picking up the phone and talking to a dear friend
- Buying myself a bunch of flowers
- Eating a bunch of grapes
- Trying out a new eye makeup
- Practicing yoga
- Dancing in front of a keep fit dance video

You get one shot at this life and it doesn't have to be drudgery. Stop making yourself do things that you don't even enjoy anymore and give yourself twenty minutes a day to do something that you want to do. You have to rediscover the ideal you and you will never do that while you are codependent. Your life doesn't revolve around the life of someone else. It may intertwine with the life of someone else, but each person is an island and that island allows for fun sometimes, as well as duty.

Look now at the definition of codependence. This comes from Psychology Today.

"Broadly speaking, in dysfunctional helping relationships, one person's help supports (enables) the other's underachievement, irresponsibility, immaturity, addiction, procrastination, or poor mental or physical health."

If that is how you see yourself now, it's time to change your way of thinking. Of course, you feel that you need to support your loved ones, but the difference is that a codependent person is willing to put up with behavior that is contrary to their wellbeing. That's not only unhealthy, but it doesn't win you any brownie points with the person you make that sacrifice for. Stop it in its tracks by learning to love yourself.

Conclusion

Over the course of this book, we have looked at all kinds of codependent relationships because it's time to stand your own ground and to be the best person you can be. You will win admiration for your honesty and for being caring enough to discuss problems, rather than pretending that your problems don't matter. I have worked with people who suffer from codependency for some years and it never fails to amaze me how pleased these people are when they break the mold and step beyond it.

"I did something for myself today" one lady told me after having looked after her mother for the past 15 years. She had practically given up on life and her mother made no effort to make her feel she had any value at all. In fact, she has moved on and is now able to care for her mother but also care for herself. It isn't selfish. It's human and it's what makes you more complete as a person.

Yet another client lives with a drunk. When they were eventually able to sit down and talk, she was able to encourage him into a program that helped him toward being sober. She was also able to start liking who she was and enjoying her time with her family more than she had for years. She didn't have to make excuses for him anymore. She didn't have to fear the repercussions anymore because she took her stand and her remorseful husband made the changes that he needed to make.

Don't enable people who do not try to improve their lives. Don't put yourself down for not being who they want you to be. Be proud of who you are. That's the most valuable gift you can ever give anyone in the world. Kenny is proud of his wife for her strength of character, whereas in the past, he felt ashamed of what he was doing to her and to the way in which she viewed her life.

There is much happiness to be had after codependence. If you really want to get beyond it, this book holds all the clues. All you need to do is take the steps that are outlined in the book and you will gradually find your way back to health again and back to a healthy state of mind where you appreciate yourself and set boundaries that help others to respect you. This book was written with a lot of emotion because this is a very emotional subject to me and to the men and women I have had to deal with over the years who suffered from the effects of codependency. When you learn to move on and to lay down what are acceptable boundaries, you help everyone – including that person who may have begun to take you for granted.

Bonus!

Thank you again for downloading this book! Please click the following link on ebook version to retain your bonus:

Mindful Codependency before Cure

I hope this book was able to help you get some value you were seeking for.

Finally, if you enjoyed this book, then I'd like to ask you for a favor, **would you be kind enough to leave a review for this book on Amazon?** It'd be greatly appreciated!

Please join us on Facebook

Thank you and good luck!